Scanning the Horizon

Using Organizational Data
to Prevent Abuse and Neglect of People
with Intellectual Disabilities

Scanning the Horizon

Using Organizational Data
to Prevent Abuse and Neglect of People
with Intellectual Disabilities

by Steve Baker and Amy Tabor

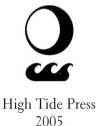

High Tide Press
2005

Published by High Tide Press, Inc.
101 Hempstead Place, Joliet, Illinois 60433

Baker, Steve and Tabor, Amy, Scanning the Horizon: using
organizational data to prevent abuse and neglect of people with
intellectural disabilities / by Steve Baker and Amy Tabor
2nd. Edition 2018

ISBN 1-892696-34-7

HighTidePress.com

Printed in the United States of America

Second Edition

Also by Steve Baker and Amy Tabor:
Human Rights Committees: Keeping Organizations on Course

In Appreciation

To Art Dykstra, for the vision to support
this and other such projects.

To Dave Hingsburger, for a life of advocacy
on behalf of others.

To Nancy Ray, for showing how prevention
is more than reporting.

To Dick Sobsey, for his quiet outrage
that keeps these fires burning.

To Jack King, for unlocking the secrets
of the Bat Cave.

Table of Contents

Dog Fox Field
by Les Murray

*The test for feeblemindedness was, they had to make up a sentence
using the words dog, fox, and field.*
                                        –"Judgment at Nuremburg"

These were no leaders, but they were first
into the dark on Dog Fox Field:

Anna who rocked her head, and Paul
who grew big and yet giggled small,

Irma who looked Chinese, and Hans
who knew his world as a fox knows a field.

Hunted with needles, exposed, unfed,
this time in their thousands they bore sad cuts

for having gaped, and shuffled, and failed
to field the lore of prey and hound

they then had to thump and cry in the vans
that ran while stopped in Dog Fox Field.

Our sentries, whose holocaust does not end,
they show us when we cross into Dog Fox Field.

Scanning the Horizon
Using Organizational Data
to Prevent Abuse and Neglect of People
with Intellectual Disabilities

Part 1
Storms on the Horizon

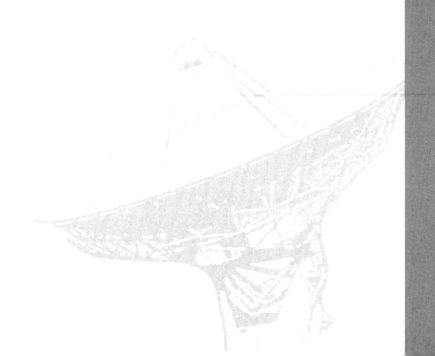

Severe Weather Watches

On August 28, 1990, a major, late-season tornado struck the small farming community of Plainfield, Illinois, scraping the ground clear for nearly seventeen miles and taking twenty-eight lives in less than five minutes. In the finger-pointing that ensued, much was made of the fact that the tornado warning sirens did not sound off until after the tornado had passed. The reality was that people were caught off guard and did not have time to take cover from the storm.

For those living in a zone known as "tornado alley," the April to August tornado season brings a lot of confusion. Each time the television beeps, announcing the arrival of a text line of weather information at the bottom of the screen, people have to go through the same mental gymnastics. Which is it–a watch or a warning that means trouble?

In the parlance of the National Weather Service, a "watch" means that current conditions favor the formation of troublesome weather. On a hot summer day, most people go about their normal routine but alter their behavior if a strong cold front approaches. If the sky in the west is starting to turn that funny green, or if the weather map on the television displays reddish/orange blobs to the west, there is a heightened sense of awareness. People stay a little closer to home, take down the patio umbrella, clean the downspouts of debris, and generally "batten down the hatches" in an effort to minimize impending storm damage.

A "warning" indicates that troublesome weather is already here. Once the storm warning sirens go off, there is little to be done but decide if it is time to locate the emergency supplies, seek shelter, or grab the camcorder and go outside to witness the awesome event. The storm has arrived; damage repair and clean-up are the next order of business.

Organizations committed to reducing abuse and neglect of vulnerable people live in a perpetual "tornado alley." But, unlike bad weather, there is no single season; the potential for abuse and neglect is ever present. And, the warnings often come too late. The damage is done. Someone has been injured. Emergency response procedures go into effect and organizational damage control begins.

When organizations learn how to recognize "watch" conditions, the situations in which trouble is more likely to arise, they have a chance to mitigate, lessen, or prevent entirely injury or neglect of the people they serve. Unlike the weather, the environment in an organization can be changed. We can alter practices to focus on prevention strategies that minimize danger and maximize choice and independence.

Scanning the Horizon is a tool that offers specific steps organizations can take to establish their own organizational radar that identifies the watch conditions. The process begins by honestly assessing the organizational climate, and using relevant data to locate the areas and conditions under which abuse and neglect are more likely to develop.

This management tool is based on analysis of substantiated cases of abuse by leading practitioners in the field. Tempered by the authors' collective half-century of experience, it guides the user in extracting data through a number of assessments, and produces a profile that examines two major areas: people supported and paid staff. Once developed, this profile will assist human service agencies to better address issues that focus on preventative measures, rather than reactionary, after-the-fact strategies. When these indicators are regularly monitored, the radar system continually alerts the organization to approaching issues of abuse and/or neglect of vulnerable people.

A History of Services

A person who is compelled to study the deplorable living conditions once endured by people with intellectual disabilities can learn a great deal about "man's inhumanity to man." Within the last century, the most profound examples are found in the evils of World War II and The Holocaust. A book entitled *Ordinary Men* (Farrar Strauss & Giroux, 1992) is a sterling reference on this subject.

It is now well known that among the earliest victims of the Nazi regime were people with intellectual disabilities. Entire German institutions were emptied to further their experiments in racial purity. Thousands of people took the "feeble-mindedness" test, attempting to construct a sentence using the words "dog," fox" and "field." Those who failed were put to death. The poem, "Dog Fox Field," by Les Murray (Farrar Strauss & Giroux, 1992) is a solemn remembrance of powerless people everywhere.

In 1941 and 1942, the German legions swept through the Baltic States and into Russia, apparently on the way to a swift capture of Moscow and perhaps Stalin himself. The rapid advances created logistical problems for the conquerors in managing and policing the additions to the Third Reich. Battalions of "Order Police" were hastily drafted, trained and deployed. The actions of these killing squads will live forever in infamy, as the horrors of Dog Fox Field became The Final Solution–death for millions of individuals. Yet, before the war, these monsters were ordinary people–the mailman, storeowner, craftsman, factory worker or farmer. These regular members of the community became convinced of the necessity for, and the correctness of their actions, carrying out crimes against humanity on a scale never before recorded. Although the duty may have been distasteful, it was deemed necessary. They did not, at the time, believe that they were doing anything wrong.

On this side of the Atlantic, people with Intellectual disabilities were warehoused in institutions, a great social nightmare of which most people outside of the profession remained blissfully unaware. The story of those times was captured by Mary Chapin Carpenter on her widely acclaimed "Stones in the Road" record album (Why Walk Music, 1994). She composed and performed an unassuming, yet powerful song entitled "John Doe No. 24." It tells the 1945 story of a young man who found himself caught up in the juggernaut of the system for people with intellectual disabilities. Because he was deaf and unable to speak, he could not convince anyone that he was not "feeble-minded." The song and his story caught the attention of *Springfield Journal-Register* reporter Dave Bakke, whose investigation resulted in the book, *God Knows His Name: The True Story of John Doe No. 24* (Southern Illinois University Press, 2000). While the work is not without flaws, it remains a moving documentary of life in large, state-operated institutions from their heyday in the 1940s and 1950s through their decline, kicking and screaming, into the new millennium.

It is a sad fact that closed doors and high walls give license to the worst humanity has to offer. Life in the state institutions was bleak and featureless; the time between daybreak and lights out was usually broken only by fights, meals and toilet times. "Patients" were subjected to medical experiments without consent and predation from every direction. This brutality was accepted, even expected, by society.

Interestingly enough, the language of the day spoke of "asylums," where the unfortunate could find solace from the stresses of daily living, which, presumably, they were unable to bear. The institution also provided the public with insulation from the truth. Typically located outside of small towns, asylums not only limited big city stressors but limited public scrutiny as well. With few exceptions, notably Burton Blatt's *Christmas in Purgatory* (Allyn & Bacon, 1966), media coverage portrayed benign scenes of pastoral calm that, however contrived, were effective at limiting the anxiety of the viewer.

Institutional change began gathering momentum in the 1960s as the John Does in the United States began to be noticed. In 1968, administrators at Bridgewater State Hospital in Massachusetts invited reporters to their facility to document what they believed to be progressive, humane programs for people committed there. The institution housed people with intellectual disabilities, many of whom were also charged with criminal offenses. The resulting film, *Titticut Follies,* had a very short exhibition life because of the public outrage that greeted its introduction on television. The premise was an inmate talent show, but the film also documented behind-the-scenes activities. It featured inmates performing everyday tasks in the bleakest of environments, urged on by uncaring staff members. The State of Massachusetts promptly went to court to block any future showing of the conditions at Bridgewater. The court order expired in the late 1990s, and copies of the compelling expose became available. This film is truly a "must see" for any serious student of the history of institutional abuse.

In 1972, journalist Geraldo Rivera and an investigative film crew used a "borrowed" key to unlock a back entrance to the Willowbrook State School on Staten Island. Inside, they discovered the horrors of mistreatment and the deplorable conditions afforded to the innocent children with intellectual disabilities committed there. The resulting footage was drastically different from the fluff piece completed earlier that showed well-dressed children in brightly colored rooms engaging in meaningful activities.

More recently, video footage has helped the federal government gain insights into service delivery problems. The Center for Medicaid Services (CMS) has used hidden cameras to document mistreatment in intermediate care facilities (ICFs). The pictures show average direct support workers taunting and injuring the people in their care. These injustices, though still far too prevalent, are now less easily hidden behind institutional walls.

Deinstitutionalization was introduced in the 1970s as an effort to improve conditions for people with intellectual disabilities. Regulators and professionals began down-sizing institutional populations and allowing the introduction of concepts like "least restrictive environment," "active treatment" and "age appropriateness." The barriers are a little lower now, and they are located more and more often in "the community" where people with disabilities now live in smaller, home-like settings. In 1988, for the first time, more money was spent nationally on community-based services for people with intellectual disabilities than for services in public and private institutions. By the year 2000, the ratio of community to institutional spending exceeded three to one (Braddock, 2003). Despite these encouraging numbers, the data actually show very little improvement in the abuse and neglect arena. The Health Care Financing Administration/Center for Medicaid Services look-behind surveys of the 1980s and 1990s helped to make it crystal clear that the problems of abuse and neglect do not vary in proportion to living unit size or location. There appears, in fact, to be little or no relationship (Ray, 2000).

It is incumbent on all of us to refuse to let atrocities from institutional life be reborn in the private sector.

Organizational Responses

Organizational responses to the pervasiveness of abuse and neglect have traditionally focused on politically visible "fixes." These
solutions are highly dependent on the establishment of paper
trails. They result in thick policy and procedural manuals filled
with the latest abuse and neglect definitions and related employee
discipline actions. While it may be argued that some organizations
instituted prevention planning some time ago, a careful review of
typical "prevention" plans tends to reveal an emphasis on investigative techniques, interrogation skills, crime scene preservation
and the re-training of staff. These efforts focus mainly on after-the-
fact responses that feature a great emphasis on behind-coverage.

One of the challenges agencies must face is transitioning from
policies based on "zero tolerance" to programs that truly focus on
prevention. The popularity of zero tolerance policies lies in the fact
that they promote a political position, since the implied "get
tough" approach plays well in the media and with financial

donors. It also seems to reassure relatives that their loved one will be in a safer environment. Zero tolerance, however, only ensures that people will be "dealt with" after the fact, once it is too late.

In actual practice, zero tolerance tends to create a whole series of problems. The policy pits employees against management, and fosters a culture that is defined by the reluctance to report abuse. It encourages the growth of fear and resentment among employees who fear that they may be treated unfairly–terminated, placed on an offender registry and/or subjected to criminal prosecution (MacNamara, 2000). The stern attitudes reflected in the manuals and the zero tolerance policies remain popular. Nevertheless, the very existence of such reactive plans is the first of our severe weather watches.

Every effective prevention program starts with positive relationships. It recognizes that we are all "ordinary men and women" and that abuse is possible any time a power differential exists between two or more people. Effective prevention is born of knowing and trusting others and is nourished by the quality of those relationships. Scanning the Horizon helps human service agencies nurture those relationships by setting up an effective internal radar screen.

Part 2
Scanning the Organization

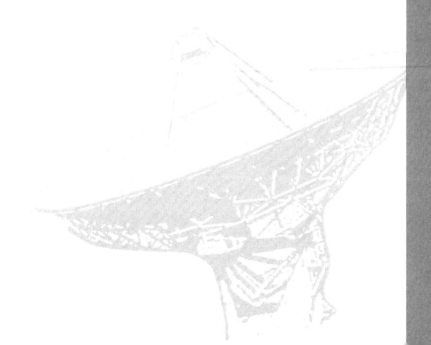

Before Starting the Assessment

Scanning the Horizon is a risk assessment tool that helps to collect organizational data in a way that expedites the identification of antecedents to abuse and/or neglect. The first step, the Tolerance Scale, will array some subjective data that will help later in the process. (See Table 1 on pages 20 and 21.)

Although "common sense" is too often anything but that, a growing body of research (Weick and Sutcliffe, 2001 and Gladwell, 2005) suggests that our "gut feelings," those instant impressions we sometimes form, can be astonishingly accurate in assessing a situation even when the objective data points in the opposite direction. The responses on the Tolerance Scale serve the same purpose.

The responses can be analyzed in three ways.

- The more items checked in the Occurs column, the greater the immediate problem.
- The number of items with a check in the Occurs column will

provide some insight on the scale of day-to-day staff behavior in your area of responsibility.

• The type and severity of items in the Occurs column relative to those in the Does Not Occur column will help to define the individualized probes as you develop an agency radar screen.

Anonymous surveys can encourage openness and frankness that might not occur otherwise. In addition, if a position title is indicated on the form, some interesting comparative data might become available.

Creating an Agency Radar Screen

The radar screen is designed to expand the subjective impressions identified in the Tolerance Scale. It examines organizational data, testing it for the presence of antecedents that your agency has identified as potential precursors of abuse and/or neglect.

A scan (or assessment) of your organization's "horizon" involves probing each of twenty *key indicators*. This is accomplished when you:

• Develop *operational definitions* to test for the presence of risk factors.
• Identify *data sources*.
• Graphically display the results on *data sheets*. (Graphs may prove helpful, too. See Table 6 on page 46.)

The Recommended Resources in each section provide additional information and inspiration to enhance the assessment process.

Key Indicators are enumerated for each of two major domains: People Supported and Paid Staff. These key indicators are fairly universal and should be recognizable as issues of significant concern to professionals, parents and key stakeholders. They define the basic conditions that should function as storm watches–the blips on the organizational radar. It is important to probe all of these indicators during an assessment whenever possible. The next two sections describe how to customize the instrument.

Operational Definitions are the warning signs–the actual behaviors, conditions or situations–that define the presence or absence of an area of concern. Although the Tolerance Scale in Table 1 lists several issues, they are simply suggestions. This exercise permits "customization" to fit the needs and culture of the organization. While you may find many of the sample definitions to be very usable, it is unlikely that the entire list will apply in every case. Therefore, you are encouraged to select the most "fitting" operational definition–the one that ensures that the data you collect accurately reflects your organization's current reality. This exercise is well worth some extra effort. Meaningful data will truly indicate the degree to which any of the risk factors are present.

In developing the operational definitions, it is important to keep the following in mind.

- Definitions must be clear and consistently applied.
- Factors must be measurable.
- Language must be specific, not ambiguous.
- Definitions must allow an absolute determination of the presence or absence of a condition.
- Only one operational definition can be selected for each key factor to ensure that the same element will be measured by multiple people.

As you are designing the assessment tools, be as specific as possible at this stage of the planning so everyone concerned agrees on exactly what will be measured. For example, when an agency examines "unhealthy overtime," it should define specifically what that means in terms of hours or frequency, or what makes sense organizationally. It may define "unhealthy overtime" as having a second full-time job somewhere else. This operational definition equips the agency to determine clearly:

- Whether a person has another job
- How many hours per week he or she works, and
- If that other job meets (or does not meet) the standard established for the presence of "unhealthy overtime."

Data Sources will vary among organizations. They are as unique as the organization and can be altered to fit individual situations. The descriptions provided in the sample worksheets are meant to aid, not prescribe. (See Table 3 on pages 34 and 35, and Table 4 on pages 41, 42 and 43.) Many avenues within the organization can serve as data sources: human resource records and statistics; staffing schedules; person supported statistics; social histories; nursing and medical records; person supported and staff interviews; general agency knowledge; and active and engaged management. The informal communication channels, or agency "grapevine," should never be ignored because that is where widely trusted, though often unreliable, information circulates.

The "radar screen" or **Organizational Profile** emerges once the following steps have been taken.
- Complete the assessment process, or scan.
- Plot the resulting data on data sheets.
- Evaluate all 20 key indicators.

Any gathering storms clouds are plain to see on this visual representation of potential high-risk areas for abuse and/or neglect. Administrators are now equipped to deal with rising threats before damage is done.

The Appendices contain sample forms for defining, collecting and analyzing the data. They are designed to aid you in developing a radar screen that reflects the unique nature of your organization.

The Tolerance Scale

The Tolerance Scale on pages 20 and 21 is provided as a guide. You may choose to customize it. Read each statement and consider whether the issue probably would or would not occur in your organization. Place a check mark in the appropriate column beside each item. Total the number of checks in each column. Use the suggestions that begin on page 15 to analyze the results before moving on to the scan, or assessment, of the organization.

Note: The exercise will prove most valuable if it is completed in a spirit of candor. Responses should not reflect what should or should not occur, but rather, "It can happen here."

Table 1. The Tolerance Scale

Occurs	Does Not Occur		Issue
		1	Staff doing her/his own laundry at the group home.
		2	Staff member embarrassing a person supported in front of his peers.
		3	Staff conducting personal errands while on the job.
		4	Staff yelling at a person supported.
		5	Staff not running programs.
		6	Staff making a medication error–wrong person, wrong dose.
		7	Staff member pulling on a person supported's elbow.
		8	Staff member using an ATM card belonging to a person supported.
		9	Staff member moving the clock hands to make it seem like bedtime.

Table 1. The Tolerance Scale (continued)

10	Staff entertaining friends while on the job.	
11	Staff bringing children to work.	
12	Staff withholding dinner because a person has been "bad."	
13	Staff arguing with each other in front of persons supported.	
14	Staff not collecting program data.	
15	Staff using profanity towards a person supported.	
16	Staff falling asleep on the job.	
17	Staff car being washed by client.	
18	Staff using alcohol while on duty.	
19	Staff retaliating physically.	
20	Staff failing to puree food per special diet order or pureeing everyone's food.	
	Totals	

Conducting the Scan

1. **Decide who should conduct the assessment.** There is not one right person or persons. Often, a number of people in an agency could fulfill the role of reviewer. Staff who administer quality assurance, program evaluation, staff development and similar functions are the most logical choices. People who are knowledgeable and experienced in many of the items being assessed are more apt to produce an accurate assessment. Objectivity, impartiality, confidentiality and tact are also important traits for reviewers. (In some instances, a team of internal reviewers may be more helpful. But, it may also prove helpful to include self-advocates on the assessment team.)

2. **Choose the environment.** Each agency or program site has unique characteristics that warrant special consideration. A key decision is how closely to "zoom" into the organization. When in doubt, administrators may see better results by reviewing a smaller,

rather than larger, area. This ensures that the data are easily observable and definable. Once data have been collected for individual sites across the organization, they can be combined to provide an overall Organizational Profile.

3. Decide when and how often to conduct the assessment. The assessment process should not be rushed; however, it is important to complete it in a defined period of time so that a "single point in time" snapshot can be taken. If the process is too drawn out, some data may become stale. Even worse, interventions may come too late. This initial assessment or "snapshot" must serve as a baseline for future assessments so agency benchmarks can be established. Each agency should determine for itself how frequent both the assessment and the re-evaluation of past benchmarks and goals will be.

For example, some agencies will benefit from completing this process annually, while others will want to monitor it more closely, perhaps quarterly or even monthly. Areas perceived to be at high risk should, of course, draw more frequent attention. (Remember, while tracking severe weather, meteorologists update their reports often.) Using a random or representative sampling method could also be useful.

4. Identify data collection sources. Data can be extracted from a number of sources and then analyzed. The sources suggested here (in Table 3 and Table 4) correlate with each of the operational definitions for the key indicators. The language used here is generic, so your agency's interpretation should include terms that are consistent with the agency. (For example, "behavior plans" may be referred to as "self-improvement plans" instead.) The blank worksheets in Appendix A and Appendix B will aid you in this process. The goal is to provide consistency so everyone knows what is being measured. Customizing is very appropriate as long as it maintains or strengthens the integrity of the inquiry.

Using the models provided in Appendix C and Appendix D, create two spreadsheets: People Supported and Paid Staff. It may be desirable to use unique individual identifiers (person supported or employee ID numbers, for example) and not actual names. This serves to protect the confidentiality of the individuals being assessed. Create data sheets for each site to be reviewed, and code them by site. A quick refernce guide may be helpful once you have identified each operational definition for each key indicator. (See Appendix E.)

5. Train the reviewers. Reviewers must be coached about how to conduct this assessment. Once trained properly, a reviewer should:

- Understand the roles of observer and data collector
- Know how to conduct the assessment as unobtrusively as possible in order to avoid overtly interacting with staff and people supported
- Have a thorough understanding of the operational definitions
- Know how to score the presence or absence of a key indicator in a way that is consistent with the intent
- Understand the reviewer's role as mandated reporter in the event he or she observes something reportable.

Training topics may also include: confidentiality, observation skills, agency values, and effective feedback techniques.

6. Inform people, families, staff and board members. Key stakeholders should be informed that an organizational assessment on service delivery effectiveness is being conducted and that their cooperation is needed. It might also be helpful to let them know that the overall results of the survey will be shared at the conclusion of the assessment process.

7. Schedule site visits. When visiting sites for data collection, reviewers should schedule and announce their arrival in most instances. The agency should send reviewers in numbers that will not create a critical shortage in any department or program, but will provide sufficient manpower to create a "single point in time" organizational snapshot. Having too many observers will compromise the integrity of the data by altering, however briefly, the environment and the daily rhythm of the site. The length of visits will vary according to environments and the reviewer's level of confidence.

8. Record and compile data. Reviewers should complete two data sheets for each site visit–one for people supported and one for paid staff. To begin, record the presence of a characteristic by placing a "1" in the appropriate box. Use one row for each person assessed and one column for each key indicator. (Using the number 1–not an X or a check mark–is best. It allows for calculations in spreadsheets as well as data display in graphs and charts.) If the characteristic is not present, do not record anything. Total each row and column as shown on the sample data sheet in Table 2.

9. Interpret the data. Once the data have been plotted on the data sheets and/or displayed in graph format, it will become clear where the significant issues that you have defined are clustered. Generally speaking, the larger the cluster, the greater the danger in the area surveyed. Please note, however, that it would be a mistake to ignore the presence of a single point or single person indicator. Each of these elements can be analyzed to provide insight. Any element, person or site that shows up over 50 percent of the time probably should receive significant and prompt attention.

In Table 2 on page 27, P-1 (History of Abuse and/or Neglect) and P-5 (Behavioral Issues) appear to be blips on the radar screen with 100 percent of the sample sharing those characteristics. Data points also appear for Person 144 quite a bit more often than for the others. The intent is not to single people out (people supported or paid staff) as "troublemakers" who need to be dealt with. Rather, the goal is to gather data indicating an alert for potential concern.

Caveats: The data collected from these assessments are extremely sensitive and personal. It should be treated with the utmost confidentiality. Misuse can easily contribute to "labeling" individuals, including staff, thus creating a high-risk situation where one might not have existed or stigmatizing an otherwise conscientious staff person. Completing this assessment will be a complex task, but the results–the ability to recognize trends and possibly prevent abuse and/or neglect in the lives of people supported–is well worth the effort.

Table 2. Sample Data Sheet: Main Street Services (MSI) People Supported

MSI Person Supported	P-1	P-2	P-3	P-4	P-5	P-6	P-7	P-8	P-9	P-10	Total
23	1				1						2
144	1	1		1	1	1					5
105	1				1			1			3
97	1				1						2
Total	4	1	0	1	4	1	0	1	0	0	12

NOTE: Using a number to identify a person supported allows for greater anonymity.

27

The Scan: People Supported

The best of current services and support strategies operate from a "person-centered" base. Effective future planning is built upon the understanding that each individual receiving services brings with him or her a personal history filled with good and bad experiences within a context of current-life circumstances. Person-centered supports begin with the person supported and expand outward to meet individual needs and conditions. This permits the individual to make more choices, become more independent and, hopefully, more confident. As a result, he or she is better equipped to resist abuse and exploitation.

Therefore, "the people we support come first" is a sentiment that both informs and drives the radar system concept. The assessment begins with the examination of ten personal elements. (See Table 3 on pages 34 and 35.)

(P-1) History of Abuse and/or Neglect

Research suggests (McCartney & Campbell, 1988) that service users with existing personal histories of abuse, neglect or exploitation are more likely to become victims of abuse, neglect or exploitation again. Sobsey (1994) suggests that as many as 81 percent of people with intellectual disabilities have been subjected to major physical or sexual assault. As many as 83 percent of this group have been victimized more than once and 50 percent more than ten times. The risk level for people with intellectual disabilities runs up to five times that of the general population.

(P-2) Reputation

An AAMR study (McCartney & Campbell, 1988) also suggests that people with bad reputations are more likely to become victims of abuse and/or neglect than those without such reputations. People known as "bad actors" often have this unfortunate information enshrined in their "permanent records," which can be exacerbated by agency gossip. The reaction of others to this characterization is to expect trouble, an expectation that too often becomes a self-fulfilling prophecy.

(P-3) Involved Medical Care

Today, staff are performing many regular medical support procedures that were once the job of nursing staff in institutional environments. Many of these activities have significant aversive elements that tend to encourage staff to take shortcuts or ignore them altogether. Thus, people receiving services, who routinely require involved medical care, are more likely to become victims of abuse and neglect (Ray, 2000).

(P-4) Involved Personal Care

People with intellectual disabilities often require additional support for personal care routines. Research suggests that service users who require involved personal care are also more likely to be victims of abuse and/or neglect, probably for many of the same reasons as involved medical care (Ray, 2000). Probes of this element focus on providing support in showering, toileting, personal hygiene, the subsequent changing of soiled clothing/linens, and other hygienic issues.

(P-5) Behavioral Issues/Plans

McCartney & Campbell (1988) also suggest that people who have active behavioral issues are particularly at risk for abuse and/or neglect. People at risk can be identified by the presence of plans for the management of behaviors, incident reports, workers' compensation statistics, employee complaints and similar types of records. People using psychotropic medications for "behaviors" or symptoms of mental illness should also be included (Dosen, 2004).

(P-6) Fiscal Vulnerability

Theft is a perpetual problem in congregate living situations as evidenced by complaints from service users and their parent/guardians. Individuals with easily accessible cash, large paychecks, money in the bank, designer clothing, electronic equipment and other desirable items are at an increased risk for theft by other service users, staff or unknown persons.

(P-7) Empowerment

People with intellectual disabilities have historically been members of a group without significant political, economic, social or personal power. Traditional plans have maintained the power imbalances through emphasis on compliance with the "commands" or "demands" of staff without much regard for individual efforts toward self-determination. "Non-compliance" is defined in many organizations as a maladaptive behavior. Attempts by staff to enforce their will often lead to power struggles between staff and people receiving services. These struggles can result in abuse of and injury to all involved. Service users who lack self-protection training or experiences are at an especially great risk of abuse and/or neglect (Reynolds, 2001). It is these power imbalances that are at the heart of the self-advocacy movement. For more information on the movement, see the materials listed in the "Resources" section.

(P-8) Down Time

Idle hands are indeed the devil's workshop. Among the strengths of community-based supports is the opportunity to be involved in more meaningful activities that increase the value of an individual's position in the fabric of the community. Inadequate scheduling for individuals can create abundant unstructured "down time" in which it is easy to revert to institutional patterns of behavior. These situations serve as breeding grounds for abuse and/or neglect (McCartney & Campbell, 1988).

(P-9) Satisfaction

Satisfaction is a basic expectation of quality supports. For purposes of this discussion, satisfaction is defined as including ways in which to comment on conditions and reasonably expect a response. People who feel trapped in their situations are far more likely to indulge in maladaptive techniques to gain attention for their issues than individuals who have effective outlets.

(P-10) Individual Service Plans

The individual service plan is the single most important planning document for people receiving services. Formally, it details the goals and objectives set for an upcoming time period. Informally, it introduces an individual to the staff who will be responsible for providing services and supports. Well-constructed, person-centered plans increase the individuals' opportunities to direct their own lives. Incomplete, inaccurate, inappropriate and/or out-of-date plans can be indicators of a culture in which the individual is not recognized as very important. Furthermore, the substandard plan does not accurately reflect the current issues in the life of the person it is designed to support. In either case, it hinders the development of critical interpersonal relationships.

Table 3. Sample Worksheet: Main Street Services (MSI) Operational Definitions for People Supported

	Key Indicator	MSI Operational Definitions	MSI Data Sources
P-1	History of Abuse, Neglect or Exploitation	Person has been victim of abuse, neglect or exploitation	Knowledge of person; incident reports; self-reporting; social histories
P-2	Reputation	Person viewed as "difficult" or "bad"	Knowledge of person; staff interviews; housemate interviews; pre-existing behavior plans
P-3	Involved Medical Care	Person requires a high level of medical care	Knowledge of person; staff interviews; nursing report; individual service plan
P-4	Involved Personal Care	Person requires a high level of personal care assistance	Knowledge of person; staff interviews; individual service plan
P-5	Behavioral Issues	· Person has "behavior plan" · Person uses psychotropic medications · Person has been the perpetrator of abuse · Person involved in property damage	QMRP/case manager statistics; copies of behavior plans; property damage; agency-wide committee minutes; medication records; pharmacy records; nursing reports; medical databases

Table 3. Sample Worksheet: Main Street Services (MSI) Operational Definitions for People Supported (continued)

P-6	Fiscal Vulnerability	· Person has significant cash/property on site · Person earns large paycheck · Person has easy access to money	Knowledge of person; financial records; agency statistics; active and engaged management
P-7	Empowerment	· Person has not been involved in individual empowerment efforts/training · Presence of "compliance" training programs	Knowledge of person; service plans
P-8	Down Time	Person spends large amounts of time not engaged in meaningful activities	Active and engaged management; individual schedules; staff interviews
P-9	Satisfaction	Person indicates dissatisfaction with services	Person supported feedback; statistics; individual service plans; guardian surveys
P-10	Individual Service Plan	· Person's service plan is outdated, incomplete, or inappropriate · Little progress on goals	QMRP/case manager statistics; random record reviews

The Scan: Paid Staff

People with intellectual disabilities are, literally, at the mercy of the staff who are paid and assigned to support them. While these employees are the backbone of every agency, in the United States they are all too often individuals who are lacking in both economic and social resources. As a result, agencies often encounter an array of staff issues that impact job performance. This radar system focuses most specifically on the non-degreed professional who has direct contact responsibilities for the people supported, even though other employee groups may be surveyed with this instrument as well. Quality of life indicators for people receiving supports and services are often a direct result of both positive and negative interactions with direct service professionals.

The term "direct service professional" will not typically include administrative or other support staff. In addition, employee candidates with conviction records and/or who have who have been terminated for abuse/neglect in other areas should be discovered during pre-employment screenings, so, they are not contemplated in this scale. (See Table 4 on pages 41 through 43.)

(S-1) Staff Vulnerability
Hiring good staff is one of the most important actions an agency takes. A recurring theme in cases of confirmed abuse and/or neglect is the staff member who is beset by excessive personal stressors that can decrease his or her ability to cope with the additional demands of challenging job situations (Ray, 2000). Staff "brittleness" is a potential indicator of vulnerability to additional stressors (MacNamara, 2000). For example, staff members who have excessive personal (non-work related) demands placed on them by others during work hours are more likely to perform poorly.

(S-2) Integrity
Personal integrity is a difficult thing to measure; yet when people fail to demonstrate it, deficits become obvious. Integrity, as it is defined here, is a practice of staff demonstrating a set of values consistent with agency values. Organizational culture can play an important part in whether these lapses are tolerated–whether they are reported and dealt with, or whether they become part of "how to get along at work."

(S-3) Isolation
The contemporary group home model emphasizes scattered sites, sometimes located miles apart or miles from administrative offices. Unlike the institutional model, where help is readily available down the hall, group home workers often find no additional help available when challenging situations arise. This type of isolation can elicit a number of undesirable behaviors. Taking shortcuts that compromise individual safety and comfort, stealing, and other acts of poor judgment are easier to pull off in a home that lacks sufficient contact with supervisors, professional staff, parents and other advocates. It is important to note that staff who have been involved in abuse and/or neglect cases often report that they knew that their actions were wrong, but they did not expect to be caught, and in fact had not been caught previously (Ray, 2000).

(S-4) Competence

The purpose of staff training is to deal with a variety of situations by establishing values, teaching discrete skills and creating the basis for personal mastery. To accomplish this, community agencies employ a number of strategies–classroom training, on-the-job training, experiential activities, independent studies, outside agency training events and other education opportunities. Training often includes a variety of curriculum modules for the employee to complete, and success is often evaluated through competency-based testing at the end of the training period. Staff who fail to complete all agency training requirements are less likely to display competence when they attempt to respond to problems correctly.

One of the most important training events is practicing proactive conflict avoidance coupled with de-escalation approaches to behavior. This training teaches the new staff member how to work with people with difficult "behaviors." Without such training, the probability vastly increases that individual staff members will resort to wholly inappropriate interventions. These behaviors will very likely resemble the practices they use at home with their children or the way their parents interacted with them.

(S-5) Confidence

A direct contact staff person's ability to feel confident in his or her job is essential to good performance. This is demonstrated most clearly in positive interactions with the individuals receiving support and services. While a certain amount of uncertainty is expected at an initial employment stage, confidence should continue to grow as the person acclimates to his or her new position.

(S-6) Voice and Language

A pleasant tone of voice is something most people expect from others. It is particularly important to be aware of one's tone, volume, word choices and demeanor when working with people of limited cognitive capacity. A person who has difficulty understanding language and social interactions under the best of circumstances is more likely to draw incorrect conclusions when voices are raised or ambiguous communication is used. For example, loud, harsh or embarrassing language will usually elicit undesirable behaviors, ranging from compliance through fear to aggression in return.

(S-7) Overtime

Overtime for staff can mean an opportunity to earn additional pay. However, excessive overtime can lead the employee to feel fatigued and perhaps act mindlessly. It may also enhance the temptation to take shortcuts, not perform assigned tasks, and become irritable with people supported. Any one of these behaviors can lead to increased opportunities for abuse and/or neglect.

(S-8) Job Satisfaction

Job satisfaction is important to most employees. In some instances, dissatisfaction may stem from an employee's internal disagreement with the agency's policy that prohibits the use of punishment in response to challenging behaviors. He or she may even attribute "problem behavior" to a lack of negative consequences for that behavior. Dissatisfaction may surface in the form of frequent complaints about people, events, situations, tasks or procedures at work.

(S-9) Supervisor Relationship

One of the most important indicators of individual employee success is the relationship that person has with his or her supervisor. This relationship is critical because of the often limited face-to-face interactions in scattered site housing. If this relationship is not good when issues arise, problems can develop and put individuals who receive services at risk.

(S-10) Employee Feedback

It is well documented that employees learn and perform best when desirable behaviors are modeled for them, and then they are given the opportunity to practice the behavior and receive immediate feedback (Reid, Parsons, & Green 1989). Performance feedback is crucial to improving quality. Fortunately, any number of evaluation systems are available for employees in a human services setting. However, if feedback is not shared in a timely fashion, the staff member may lose a message needed for improvement, and the supervisor may lose the opportunity to reinforce desirable behavior. In addition to on-site feedback, the employee evaluation process can be among the most effective management tools.

Table 4. Sample Worksheet: Main Street Services (MSI) Operational Definitions for Paid Staff

Key Indicator		MSI Operational Definitions	MSI Data Sources
S-1	Vulnerability	· Staff member demonstrates poor performance and reports the reason as significant personal difficulties · Staff member makes/receives too many personal calls at work	· Active, engaged management · Supervisory relationships · Disciplinary reports · Personnel files
S-2	Integrity	· Staff member continually conducts personal business while on agency time · Staff member takes advantage of agency "consumable" resources for personal use	· Employee discipline · Staff interviews · Inventories

Table 4. Sample Worksheet: Main Street Services (MSI) Operational Definitions for Paid Staff (continued)

S-3	Isolation	· Staff member regularly works alone on shifts · Staff member has a supervisor who rarely visits · Staff member is present or involved in "unusual incident" · Staff member is present or involved in "unexplained injury"	· Staff schedules · Incident/injury reports · Payroll data · Worker's compensation data
S-4	Competence	· Staff member fails to complete all required training · Staff member uses punishment in response to behavioral challenges	· Staff training records · Active, engaged management
S-5	Confidence	· Staff member responds with uncertainty in dealing with challenging issues · Staff member appears "afraid" when working with person supported	· Staff surveys · Training feedback · OJT records
S-6	Voice/ Language	· Staff member regularly uses loud tone of voice when interacting with persons supported. · Eye contact by staff is minimal to non-existent · Language appears to be aimed at controlling behavior	· Active, engaged management · Staff interviews · Person supported interviews · Investigations

Table 4. Sample Worksheet: Main Street Services (MSI) Operational Definitions for Paid Staff (continued)

S-7	Overtime	· Staff member regularly works "unhealthy" amount of overtime or full time at a second job	· Staffing schedule · Sign-in sheets · Payroll data
S-8	Job Satisfaction	· Staff member regularly states negative opinions of working conditions and/or persons supported · Staff member demonstrates a negative attitude in his/her behavior	· General knowledge of staff · Staff surveys and interviews · Supervisory reports · Performance evaluations · Person supported interviews · Morale index
S-9	Supervisor Relationship	· Staff member's relationship with supervisor is characterized as "negative" · Staff member files formal or informal grievances · Staff member turnover rates	· Personnel statistics · Staff surveys · Self-reporting · Supervisory reports · Grievance reports
S-10	Employee Feedback	· Staff member did not have an evaluation completed within the last year · Staff member does not receive regular feedback on individual tasks	· Human resource statistics · Training records · Supervisory practices

A Progressive Response

Once you have identified where the issues are, how does the agency respond? At the organization depicted in Table 5 on page 46, 100 percent of the sample for a specific site has a history of abuse and/or neglect and behavioral issues. Knowing this history allows the agency to form a plan. (Table 6, also on page 46, shows an effective way to display the results of the scan.)

The first appropriate step might be completing additional proactive behavioral training with the staff. Or, the approach might start with additional staff education on the abuses historically endured by people with intellectual disabilities. Since *everyone* in this environment exhibits what has been defined as problematic behavior, an in-depth analysis of the factors maintaining that behavior would also be warranted. The analysis would not likely be essential to carrying out more effective interventions.

Table 5. Sample Data Record: Main Street Group Home

MSI Data Record					Site:	*Main Street Group Home*				
Person Supported	P-1	P-2	P-3	P-4	P-5	P-6	P-7	P-8	P-9	P-10	Totals
43	1	0	0	0	1	0	0	0	0	0	2
20	1	1	0	1	1	1	0	0	0	0	5
129	1	0	0	0	1	0	0	1	0	0	3
77	1	0	0	0	1	0	0	0	0	0	2
65	0	0	0	0	1	0	1	0	0	0	2
122	0	0	0	0	0	0	0	1	0	0	1
94	1	1	0	0	0	1	1	0	0	0	4
51	0	0	0	0	1	0	0	0	0	0	1
TOTALS	5	2	0	1	6	2	2	2	0	0	20
%	63%	25%	0%	13%	75%	25%	25%	25%	0%	0%	25%

Table 6. Sample Data Graph: Main Street Group Home

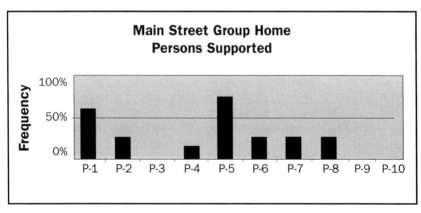

Note: In this example, P-1 and P-5 exceed the 50 percent rule.

Part 3
Reducing Vulnerability and Developing Interventions

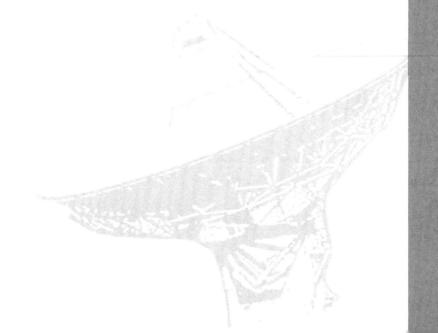

Resources for Change

At this point in the review process, the agency has created a "radar screen," or organizational profile, that indicates strength in some areas and vulnerability in others. There is now a clear indication of where to concentrate effort and resources.

"Making Your Agency Abuse-Proof," a book that should be written someday, would encompass far more than we can effectively manage in these few pages. This section does, however, offer several strategies for reducing vulnerability. It also names several resources that are helpful in developing effective interventions. It is worth noting that, despite their separate domains, many of the strategies discussed here will overlap.

Awareness is the first step. Now is the time for action.

Resources: People Supported

Supports for people can be dramatically improved without necessarily investing a great deal of tangible resources. The key is to refocus attention and action toward the higher risk areas that your agency has identified. The activities described in this section are offered both as stand-alone recommendations and as prompts to guide additional discussion.

(P-1) History of Abuse and/or Neglect
Many agencies will show multiple entries on this key indicator, reflecting the prevalence of abuse histories in the lives of people they serve and support.
- Appoint active and empowered agency human rights, behavior management and incident review committees. These committees have the ability to protect and advocate for people supported in a very proactive fashion. Trend analysis can be used to spot issues before they become larger problems. Encourage people supported to participate actively to the extent they desire.

- Increase staff training opportunities. These opportunities would include a historical perspective of the abuse and neglect of people with intellectual disabilities; signs of abuse and neglect; the nature of rights limitations as temporary measures; disability awareness; and similar issues.
- Create counseling opportunities for people in need. Given the prevalence of abuse histories in people receiving services, additional counseling opportunities may be helpful even when the incidents happened long ago. Involve social workers, mental health professionals, self-advocates and other appropriate professionals.

Recommended Resources
Christmas in Purgatory, Burton Blatt
Titticut Follies (video or DVD), Frederick Wiseman
Unforgotten: 25 Years After Willowbrook (video) Heartshare Human
  Services of New York
Circles I: Intimacy and Relationships, James Stanfield Company
Doing What Comes Naturally?, Orieda Horn Anderson
Human Sexuality Handbook: Guiding People Towards Positive
  Expressions of Sexuality, The Association for Community Living
Insight Dialog Deck and Facilitators Guide, The Hawthorne Group

(P-2) Reputation
It is not uncommon for people with intellectual disabilities to arrive in a new setting with negative reputations. Therefore, service providers need to address the following.
- Ensure that the individual service plan process includes more positive elements, similar to a resume that focuses on positive aspects rather than a confessional detailing all past "sins."
- Support people in character-building occasions to increase self-esteem that can lead to relationship enhancements.
- Emphasize the importance of confidentiality with staff.
- Reinforce with staff the dangers of "preconceived" notions through staff training experiences.

Recommended Resources
Person-Centered Planning, Mary Mercer
It's Never Too Early, It's Never Too Late: A Booklet about Personal

Futures Planning, Minnesota Governor's Planning Council on Developmental Disabilities

Read My Lips: It's My Choice, Minnesota Governor's Planning Council on Developmental Disabilities

Personal Outcome Measures, The Council on Quality and Leadership in Supports for People with Disabilities

(P-3 and P-4) Involved Medical Care and Involved Personal Care
As job descriptions in community-based organizations continue to increase job responsibilities, staff are continually being challenged in new directions. For some staff, assisting with involved medical or personal care is significantly more difficult.

- Ensure good interviewing processes. Full disclosure on job responsibilities before hiring allows potential employees to be fully aware of what they are getting into before accepting a position. (This practice may also reduce the turnover rate of your direct contact staff.)
- Use behavioral interviewing techniques when selecting staff.
- Match staff with people supported within their environment. Involve individuals who receive supports and services in the selection process when interviewing employee candidates.
- Create high quality training programs. They should include sensitivity training, non-verbal communication, procedural training that is focused on individual needs, personal preferences/styles and so on.

Recommended Resources
Behavior Description Interviewing, Tom Janz and Greg Mooney
Getting Involved in Choosing Staff, Ruth Townsley et al.
Medical Issues for Adults with Mental Retardation/Developmental Disabilities, Carl Tyler
The Ethics of Touch, Dave Hingsburger and Mary Harber
Direct Support: A Realistic Job Preview (video), Research and Training Center on Community Living

(P-5) Behavioral Issues
Without a doubt, many agencies will have concerns about the behaviors of some of the people supported. One of the most important aspects of this issue is helping the people supported and paid

staff to understand that behavior is a form of communication that is rarely driven by hostility towards others–no matter how it looks.

- Work with people supported to increase knowledge of alternate forms of self-expression.
- Increase opportunities for staff to learn about behavior as communication; use and side effects of psychotropic medications; least restrictive environments; and mental health issues.
- Develop objective measurement and display techniques for purposes of analyzing the functions of behavior (antecedent, behavior and consequence.)

Recommended Resources

Shift Happens: Making the Shift to Proactive Behavior Management, George Seuss

Functional Assessment and Intervention, James Carr and David Wilder

Antecedent Control: Innovative Approaches to Behavioral Support, James Luiselli and Michael J. Cameron

Do? Be? Do?, Dave Hingsburger

Behaviour Self, Dave Hingsburger

Don't Shoot the Dog, Karen Pryor

The Suzie Brown Intervention Maze, John Shephard

Learning to Listen: Positive Approaches and People with Difficult Behavior, Herbert Lovett

Decreasing Behavior of Persons with Severe Retardation and Autism, Richard Foxx

Increasing Behavior of Persons with Severe Retardation and Autism, Richard Foxx

Nonviolent Crisis Intervention[R] Training Program, Crisis Prevention Institute

(P-6) Fiscal Vulnerability

In an era when more people with intellectual disabilities are gaining control of their resources, it is increasingly important to be vigilant in preventing financial exploitation anywhere in the agency. For people supported who exhibit fiscal vulnerability, a series of proactive approaches can be put in place.

- Work with people supported to use keys and locks to protect their personal possessions.

- Create opportunities for individuals to access their money in an environment that balances security and individual needs.
- Develop additional fiscal training for people supported.
- Encourage people to label or mark their possessions in a respectful fashion.

Recommended Resources
Money Doesn't Grow on Trees: A Parent's Guide to Raising Financially Responsible Children, Neale S. Godfrey and Carolina Edwards
Money Smart–An Adult Education Program, Federal Deposit Insurance Corporation

(P-7) Empowerment
Many of the issues faced by people with intellectual disabilities are rooted in a desire to gain increased control over their lives. This process may pit people supported against paid staff members and result in power struggles.

- Coordinate the development of people supported in a Bill of Rights process. Instead of using the standard, annual "rights statement," create one from the individual perspective.
- Increase efforts to ensure that individuals know and understand their rights.
- Support people in presenting the issues themselves in the relevant committee discussions, such as the human rights committee, safety committee and other appropriate forums.
- Encourage the formation of self-advocacy groups, such as People First.
- Encourage individuals to exercise their right to say "no."
- Eliminate "compliance training."
- Make the environment one in which people supported, their families and staff feel comfortable talking about abuse.
- Conduct staff training about appropriate and inappropriate staff roles (mentor, advocate and teacher vs. parent, boss or maid), as well as normalization theory, age appropriateness, and related issues.
- Support people to empower themselves by providing opportunities to increase self-esteem.
- Work with people to increase their social capital networks.

Recommended Resources

Just Say Know, Dave Hingsburger
i to I, Dave Hingsburger
I Witness, Dave Hingsburger
Power Tools, Dave Hingsburger
Self-Advocates Becoming Empowered (SABE) http://www.sabe.org
Human Rights Committees: Keeping Organizations on Course,
 Steve Baker and Amy Tabor
Feel Our Freedom, Alisa Hauser Kraft
Rights Bingo (game), Colorado Ombudsman Program
The Principles and Practices of Universal Enhancement,
 Tom Pomeranz
Insight Dialog Deck and Facilitators Guide, The Hawthorne Group

(P-8) Down Time

Agencies often face the issue of the empty spots in schedules that
encourage disruptive behavior and foster inappropriate responses.
Careful attention to the daily schedules of people supported can
alleviate many of these concerns.

- Evaluate daily schedules to ensure that staffing patterns match
  the demand for services.
- Examine the person-centered planning process to make sure
  that it is being implemented effectively.
- Conduct personal preference and interest surveys to connect
  individual interests to opportunities for participation.
- Increase the availability of resources to increase individualized
  opportunities.
- Review transportation services and their availability for persons supported.
- Create a regionalized "resource activities" book that identifies cost, hours, locations, amenities and other activity-
  related information.
- Conduct staff training that encourages the importance of
  engaging people in a meaningful manner and using creativity
  to meet a person's needs.

Recommended Resources

Newspaper subscriptions
Weekend guides

Community resource directory
Parks and recreation brochures
Community centers
Tourism/convention and visitors bureau

(P-9) Satisfaction

To effectively match resources with what is important to the individual receiving services, it is best to continually assess the needs and preferences of that person.

- Use self-assessment processes to provide insight into a person's dissatisfaction.
- Conduct a consumer satisfaction process so that staff gain valuable, specific data.
- Consider using multiple methods of assessing satisfaction, perhaps using focus groups to gather feedback in a way that increases individual comfort levels.
- Encourage guardians and members of the individual's social network to provide feedback on the quality of supports and services.

Recommended Resources

The Place That Quality Built, The Council on Quality and
  Leadership in Supports for People with Disabilities
Personal Outcome Measures, The Council on Quality and
  Leadership in Supports for People with Disabilities
First, Break All the Rules, Marcus Buckingham and Curt Coffman

(P-10) Individual Service Plans

This key document aligns and links all services provided to people supported. The case manager or QMRP role is integral to the development of a personal profile that will help all staff gain insight about the person supported.

- Look to a person-centered or person-directed planning process to increase individualization of service plans.
- Encourage responsible time management practices within case management or QMRP duties.
- Reinforce the advocacy relationship between the person supported and the case manager or QMRP responsible for plan implementation.
- Implement a process of random reviews of individual progress

to identify individuals who fail to make progress on their goals. This will indicate the appropriateness of the selected goals and overall plan.

Recommended Resources

Person-Centered Planning: Helping People with Disabilities Achieve Personal Outcomes, Mary Mercer
It's Never Too Early, It's Never Too Late: A Booklet about Personal Futures Planning, Minnesota Governor's Planning Council on Developmental Disabilities
Guidebook for QMRPs, North Dakota Center for Persons with Disabilities
My Choice, Your Decision (video), Advocating Change Together
Read My Lips: It's My Choice, Minnesota Governor's Planning Council on Developmental Disabilities
Personal Outcome Measures, The Council on Quality and Leadership in Supports for People with Disabilities
National Association of Qualified Mental Retardation Professionals, www.qmrp.org (Q Notes section, especially)
Outcome Management, Art Dykstra

General Notes on Challenging Behavior

Given the predisposition within this field toward homogeneous groupings, clusters of vulnerabilities are likely to exist among the people supported. Often, at least one of these clusters will center around behavioral issues that are considered obstacles to individual growth and progress. There are a number of approaches to these issues.

Although behaviorists will cringe at the imprecise vocabulary, it remains true that behavior is maintained by two things: to get something (i.e., to make something happen) and to make something go or stay away. Attention is one of those "somethings" that is rarely available in adequate quantities to people with intellectual disabilities. Substantial research in the past few years indicates that planned attention, also known as non-contingent reinforcement (NCR), is an effective technique for reducing maladaptive behaviors. NCR techniques may be helpful in adding structure to daily routines, and in giving guidance to staff as well.

Challenging behaviors, or any behaviors for that matter, always serve some function for the individual. Identifying and understanding that function is crucial to teaching positive alternatives, as failure to do so vastly increases the risk that interventions will, in fact, reinforce the behavior in question. It is imperative, then, that staff expend a great deal of effort getting to know the person being supported.

Sometimes, problem behaviors arise simply because there is no other apparent recourse. "Pressure relief valves" for people supported may help to reduce conflict and obviate the need for "behavior plans." These include confidential contact points, warm/hot lines and structured communication channels. These options can all help relieve the stress of situations that make individuals feel trapped, and offer alternatives to confrontation.

Strong personal relationships are essential to building the trust necessary for working cooperatively and solving problems effectively. Perhaps just as important, they help direct contact staff to get past the bad reputations and troublesome personal histories, and work on meaningful objectives.

Resources: Paid Staff

It is highly unlikely that any agency can protect all of its employees from the stressors of life and the consequences of their decisions. On the other hand, it is quite possible to assist people in controlling their reactions to situations, and gaining competence and confidence at work. This also includes forming strong, productive relationships with supervisors, co-workers and the people they support every day.

(S-1) Vulnerability

In any organization, a certain number of staff members will likely be seen as especially vulnerable to even the minor ups and downs of life. This fact should probably be recognized in "boiler plate" fashion in the agency's personnel practices. It is impossible to remedy all of the world's woes, but a little flexibility in strategic places can go a long way toward minimizing conflicts between the job and the rest of a person's life.

- Foster relationships of trust between paid staff and people sup-ported. The availability of helpful attention will go a long way toward reducing problematic behavior within both groups.
- Foster relationships of trust between first line supervisors and their staff. Ensure that supervisors are available and capable of offering support to their staff.
- Examine time off policies. Consider, for example, increasing the emphasis on personal time, and making it available in relatively small increments. This might present the agency with an opportunity to decrease paid sick leave, which is typically used at the rate at which it is earned, regardless of the total amount available.
- Consider creating low-interest or no-interest loans from a small revolving fund. This has proven effective in reducing absenteeism and reducing pressure points for cash-strapped staff whose car, for example, has just blown a transmission.
- Along with everything else, an agency must see its role as advocate for better pay for its staff. It must also recognize staff members' roles as professionals, regardless of the lack of letters behind their signatures.

Recommended Resources
Bringing Out the Best in People, Aubrey Daniels
Other People's Habits, Aubrey Daniels
1001 Ways to Reward Employees, Bob Nelson
How to Recognize and Reward Employees, Donna Deeprose
The Servant Leader, James Autry
First, Break All the Rules, Marcus Buckingham and Curt Coffman
Choices: Discover Your 100 Most Important Life Choices, Shad Helmstetter

(S-2) Integrity
In areas where inventory shrinkage or time theft is detected, a number of options exist.
- Consider taking inventories at each shift change as a short-term measure. This will usually sharply decrease commodity theft.
- Ask the people supported. If that all-important, trusting relationship has been established, the people receiving services will be comfortable answering when asked what is

going on. People who feel supported will complain if they feel maltreated.

- Develop clear expectations of job performance.
- Establish consistent and busy daily routines.
- Use clear, measurable performance standards.
- Encourage the growth of a culture that ensures that many different people show up at unpredictable times. This is one of the most effective weapons available and costs little or nothing.

Recommended Resources
Outcome Management, Art Dykstra
Why Employees Don't Do What They're Supposed to Do, Ferdinand Fournies
The Exemplar Employee, Art Dykstra and Deborah Gustafson
The Ethics of Touch, Dave Hingsburger and Mary Harber

(S-3) Isolation
Except perhaps in small, campus-based programs, isolation frequently emerges as an area of concern. Isolation occurs because of the presence of opportunities for poor decision-making by the staff assigned to a given location.

- Establish a clear understanding of the factors that maintain individual behaviors. This is critical to developing interventions that teach the staff positive alternatives they find both understandable and doable.
- Create on-site training. This may be the only way staff have the opportunity to practice and receive feedback on their performance under their actual work conditions.
- Provide readily available communications with back-up resources. Even a phone consultation can go a long way toward limiting the anxiety people experience while working in an isolated setting. Again, a culture that encourages other people to stop by is critical.

Recommended Resources
Person-Centered Planning: Helping People with Disabilities Achieve Personal Outcomes, Mary Mercer
Don't Shoot the Dog, Karen Pryor
Managing People Is Like Herding Cats, Warren Bennis

(S-4) Competence

Genuine competence can limit anxiety and encourage good decision making. It can also help to build the trusting relationships that are vital to a healthy organization.

- Ensure that all staff members get to know the people supported as well as possible. Encourage participation in the development of personal sketches and individual habilitation plans that truly describe the individual as a person to be supported, not a case to be managed.
- Support staff in gaining a thorough understanding of habilitation and training plans that clearly identify the target behaviors, the desired outcomes and the ways to reach those outcomes. Provide them with opportunities to become practiced in carrying out responsibilities, and have support available when things do not go as anticipated.
- Develop on-site training with practice and feedback.
- Create staff development standards that exceed, in both quality and quantity, minimally accepted standards as set forth by state certification agencies.

Recommended Resources

Staff Management in Human Services, Dennis H. Reid, Marsha B. Parsons, and Carolyn W. Green

Developing Staff Competencies for Supporting People with Developmental Disabilities: An Orientation Handbook, James F. Gardner and Michael S. Chapman

Getting Things Done When You Are Not in Charge, Geoffrey M. Bellman

(S-5) Confidence

An inevitable offshoot of burgeoning competence is the growth of confidence. That confidence will help to make the proper responses to stressful situations automatic and positive.

- Remove obstacles to interactions between staff and people supported. This begins with removing physical barriers (nurses' stations, enclosed offices) and psychological barriers (uniforms, name badges and similar symbols of authority).
- Encourage employees who know the individuals best to develop plans for activities in which they can participate.

Avoid canned programs that make little sense to employees who are supposed to carry them out. They have little chance of being implemented properly.

- Establish supervisor work schedules that ensure maximum face-to-face interaction time with staff.
- Promote an organizational culture that is geared toward the involvement–in a deeply personal way–of all staff in helping to make everyone's life a bit better every day.

Recommended Resources
A Credo for Support (video), Norman Kunc and Emma Van der Klift, Axis Consultation
The Servant Leader, James A. Autry
The Character of Leadership, Michael Jinkins and Deborah Bradshaw Jinkins

(S-6) Voice and Language
As important an issue as tone of voice and language can be, it is one that agencies often address inadequately.

- Support people sufficiently so they feel empowered to resist coercive or overly loud language. "Non-compliance" must not be defined as a maladaptive behavior. When a person supported says "no" in appropriate situations, aggressive language is less likely to be reinforced.
- Coach staff to "act" out a role that includes appropriate verbalization. Voice coaching and "acting" lessons can provide worthwhile solutions in some situations.
- Implement agency policies and practices that discourage those things (voice, dress, behavior) that do not project respect for people supported. Reinforce those that do.

Recommended Resources
The Disney Way Fieldbook: How to Implement Walt Disney's Vision of "Dream, Believe, Dare, Do" in Your Own Company, Bill Capodagli and Lynn Jackson

(S-7) Overtime
Staff who are working multiple jobs present some of the toughest issues to solve. Because they look outside the agency for opportu-

nities to work extra hours, their work with the people supported sometimes suffers.

- Create overtime opportunities so that they are available, within reason, to staff who need them. Staff will often forgo opportunities for outside employment if they can make the same money at the agency, especially if they earn time-and-a-half pay. Making that money in fewer hours (i.e., no travel/transition time to a second job) also allows the employee more time for family and personal issues. This lessens the impact of those issues on the job. Overtime opportunities can also make the agency the "priority employer" in the mind of the employee.
- Examine work schedules to identify overtime opportunities that do not fall too closely upon other shifts, thereby minimizing back-to-back shifts. Once again, the relationship with the immediate supervisor will determine if that balance can be reached and maintained.

Recommended Resources
Outcome Management, Art Dykstra

(S-8) Satisfaction
Job satisfaction is an elusive factor that does not always correlate with job performance. It seems certain, however, that the quality of relationships with the people supported will suffer when employees are dissatisfied.

- Determine the exact nature of sources of dissatisfaction among employees.
- Reinforce the role of manager as mentor and support for staff.
- Consider job reassignments to better match employee skills with organizational needs.
- Establish the use of pressure relief valves for employees. One example is an expedited "suggestion" system that bypasses layers of bureaucracy and requires a prompt response from an upper management staff person.
- Actively participate in trade and advocacy organizations to improve overall working conditions for staff. Participation can include lobbying the legislature, participating in pooled loan programs, and receiving group membership

rates, enhanced educational opportunities, and other benefits that are attractive to employees.

Recommended Resources
First, Break All the Rules, Marcus Buckingham and Curt Coffman
Job Satisfaction: Application, Assessment, Causes and Consequences, Paul E. Spector
Frontline Supervisor's Handbook, Cindy Haworth and Mary Mercer

(S-9) Relationship with the Supervisor
The "miners' canary" of organizational health is the employee-supervisor relationship. As relationships grow stronger, most identified areas will show corresponding improvements.
- Support supervisors in knowing, understanding and supporting the people who work for them.
- Encourage supervisors to be present on the work sites, deal face-to-face with employees, and provide the support needed in tough situations.
- Examine supervisory schedules to ensure maximum presence during high-risk periods.

Recommended Resources
Managing the Unexpected, Karl Weick and Kathleen Sutcliffe
Bringing Out the Best in People, Aubrey Daniels
Why Employees Don't Do What They Are Supposed to Do, Ferdinand Fourniers
The Exemplar Employee, Art Dykstra and Deborah Gustafson

(S-10) Feedback
Regular feedback is an integral part of building the supervisory relationship. Performance on the job improves when the desired outcomes are demonstrated, opportunity for practice is given, and immediate feedback is provided.
- Evaluate the performance evaluation system to see how well it addresses the need for effective performance feedback.
- Maximize the ratio of on-site training to classroom training.

Recommended Resources:
Other People's Habits, Aubrey Daniels

Evaluation with Power: A New Approach to Organizational Effectiveness, Empowerment, and Excellence, Sandra Gray et al. *Staff Management in Human Services: Behavioral Research and Applications*, David H. Reid, Marsha B. Parsons and Carolyn W. Green

It's a Wrap!

Readers who have made it this far have, no doubt, noticed some themes.

1. Examine how well people supported, staff and supervisors know each other and determine how that can be improved.
2. Adjust staff training to include on-site opportunities with immediate feedback.
3. Do whatever it takes to improve employee-supervisor relationships.
4. Limit, where possible, the friction between the job and the employee's life outside of work.
5. Develop clear and relevant habilitation plans with extensive input from those who will carry them out.
6. Arrange for visitors, lots of visitors.

None of this is too expensive. Failing to act is.

Notes

Bakke, David. (2000). *God Knows His Name*. Carbondale, IL: Southern Illinois University Press.

Blatt, Burton, and Kaplan, Fred. (1966). *Christmas in Purgatory*. Syracuse, NY: Allyn & Bacon.

Braddock, David. (2003). *Disability at the Dawn of the 21st Century and The State of the States*. Washington, DC: American Association on Mental Retardation.

Browning, Christopher. (1992). *Ordinary Men*. New York: HarperCollins.

Capodagli, Bill, and Jackson, Lynn. (2001). *The Disney Way Fieldbook*. New York: McGraw Hill.

Dosen, Anton. (2004). The Developmental Psychiatric Approach to Aggressive Behavior among Persons with Intellectual Disabilities. *Mental Health Aspects of Developmental Disabilities,* 7 (2), 57-68.

McCartney, John R., and Campbell, Vincent A. (1988). Confirmed Abuse Cases in Public Residential Facilities for Persons with Mental Retardation: A Multi-State Study. *Mental Retardation,* 36 (6), 465-473.

McNamara, Roger. *Not Knowingly Do Harm.* [On-line]. No longer available: www.freedomfromabuse.org.

Murray, Les. (1992). "Dog Fox Field" from *Dog Fox Field: Poems.* New York: Farrar Straus & Giroux.

Ray, Nancy K. (2000). *Abuse and Neglect Prevention in Community Homes.* Presentation at Illinois American Association on Mental Retardation Conference, Collinsville, IL.

Reid, Dennis H., Parsons, Margaret B., and Green, Carolyn W. (1989). *Staff Management in Human Services: Behavioral Research and Applications.* Springfield, IL: Charles E Thomas.

Reynolds, Leigh Ann. (2001). *People With Mental Retardation and Sexual Abuse: The ARC's Q & A on People With Mental Retardation.* [On-line]. Available: www.thearc.org/faqs/Sexabuse.html (accessed July 7, 2005).

Sobsey, Dick. (1994). *Violence and Abuse in the Lives of People with Disabilities: The End of Silent Acceptance?* Baltimore: Paul H Brookes.

Weick, Carl, and Sutcliffe, Kathleen M. (2001). *Managing the Unexpected.* San Francisco: Jossey-Bass.

References

Allen, W. T. (1989). *Read My Lips: It's My Choice.* St. Paul, MN: Governor's Planning Council on Developmental Disabilities.

Anderson, Orieda Horn. (2000). *Doing What Comes Naturally? Dispelling Myths and Fallacies about Sexuality and People with Developmental Disabilities.* Homewood, IL: High Tide Press.

Autry, James A. (2001). *The Servant Leader: How to Build a Creative Team, Develop Great Morale, and Improve Bottom-Line Performance.* Roseville, CA: Prima Publishing.

Baker, Steve, and Tabor, Amy. (1999). *Human Rights Committees: Keeping Organizations on Course.* Homewood, IL: High Tide Press.

Bakke, David. (2000). *God Knows His Name*. Carbondale, IL: Southern Illinois University Press.

Bellman, Geoffrey M. (1992). *Getting Things Done When You Are Not in Charge: How to Succeed from a Support Position*. San Francisco: Berrett-Koehler.

Bennis, Warren G. (1997). *Managing People Is Like Herding Cats: Warren Bennis on Leadership*. Provo, UT: Executive Excellence.

Blatt, Burton, and Kaplan, Fred. (1966). *Christmas in Purgatory*. Syracuse, NY: Allyn & Bacon.

Braddock, David. (2003). *Disability at the Dawn of the 21st Century and The State of the States*. Washington, DC: American Association on Mental Retardation.

Brown, Gail T., et al. (1985). *Human Sexuality Handbook: Guiding People towards Positive Expressions of Sexuality*. Springfield, MA: The Association for Community Living.

Browning, Christopher. (1992). *Ordinary Men*. New York: HarperCollins.

Buckingham, Marcus, and Coffman, Curt. (1999). *First, Break All the Rules: What the World's Greatest Managers Do Differently*. New York: Simon & Schuster.

Capodagli, Bill, and Jackson, Lynn. (2001). *The Disney Way Fieldbook*. New York: McGraw Hill.

Carr, James, and Wilder, David. (1998). *Functional Assessment and Intervention: A Guide to Understanding Problem Behavior*. Homewood, IL: High Tide Press.

The Council on Quality and Leadership in Supports of People with Disabilities. (2000). *Personal Outcome Measures*. Towson, MD: Author.

The Council on Quality and Leadership in Supports of People with Disabilities. (2003). *The Place That Quality Built.* Towson, MD: Author.

Daniels, Aubrey. (2000). *Bringing Out the Best in People: How to Apply the Astonishing Power of Positive Reinforcement.* New York: McGraw-Hill.

Daniels, Aubrey. (2000). *Other People's Habits: How to Use Positive Reinforcement to Bring Out the Best in People Around You.* New York: McGraw-Hill.

Deeprose, Donna. (1994). *How to Recognize and Reward Employees.* New York: AMACOM.

Dosen, Anton. (2004). The Developmental Psychiatric Approach to Aggressive Behavior among Persons with Intellectual Disabilities. *Mental Health Aspects of Developmental Disabilities* 7 (2), 57-68.

Dykstra, Art. (1995). *Outcome Management: Achieving Outcomes for People with Disabilities.* Homewood, IL: High Tide Press.

Dykstra, Art, and Gustafson, Deborah. (1999). *The Exemplar Employee.* Homewood, IL: High Tide Press.

Dykstra, Art, Haworth, Cindy, and Williams, Timothy. (2000). *Insight Dialog Deck and Facilitators Guide: Preventing Abuse and Neglect.* Portland, OR: The Hawthorne Group International.

Fournies, Ferdinand F. (1988). *Why Employees Don't Do What They're Supposed to Do and What to Do about It.* Pine Ridge Summit, PA: Liberty House.

Foxx, Richard M. (1982). *Decreasing Behaviors of Persons with Severe Retardation and Autism.* Champaign, IL: Research Press.

Foxx, Richard M. (1982). *Increasing Behaviors of Persons with Severe Retardation and Autism.* Champaign, IL: Research Press.

Furay, Eileen M. (Ed.). (1997). *Abuse, Neglect, and People with Mental Retardation.* Worthington, OH: IDS.

Gardner, James F., and Chapman, Michael S. (1995). *Developing Staff Competencies for Supporting People with Developmental Disabilities: An Orientation Handbook.* (2nd ed.). Baltimore: Paul H. Brookes.

Godfrey, Neale S., and Edwards, Carolina. (1994). *Money Doesn't Grow on Trees: A Parent's Guide to Raising Financially Responsible Children.* Englewood Cliffs, NJ: Prentice Hall.

Gray, Sandra Trice, et al. (1997). *Evaluation with Power: A New Approach to Organization Effectiveness, Empowerment and Excellence.* San Francisco: Jossey-Bass.

Hastings, Richard P. (2002). Do Challenging Behaviors Affect Staff Psychological Well-Being? Issues of Causality and Mechanism. *American Journal on Mental Retardation* 107, 455-467.

Haworth, Cindy, and Mercer, Mary. (2004). *Frontline Supervisor's Handbook.* Minot, ND: The North Dakota Center for Persons with Disabilities.

Helmstetter, Shad. (1992). *Choices: Discover Your 100 Most Important Life Choices.* New York: Pocket Books.

Hingsburger, Dave. (1990). *i to I: Self Concept for People with Developmental Disabilities.* Mountville, PA: Vida.

Hingsburger, Dave. (1992). *I Witness: History and a Person with Developmental Disabilities.* Bear Creek, NC: Psych-Media.

Hingsburger, Dave. (1995). *Just Say Know.* Eastman, QC, Canada: Diverse City Press.

Hingsburger, Dave. (1996). *Behaviour Self.* Eastman, QC, Canada: Diverse City Press.

Hingsburger, Dave. (1998). *Do? Be? Do?* Eastman, QC, Canada: Diverse City Press.

Hingsburger, Dave. (2000). *Power Tools.* Eastman, QC, Canada: Diverse City Press.

Hingsburger, Dave, and Harber, Mary. (1998). *The Ethics of Touch: Establishing and Maintaining Appropriate Boundaries in Service to People with Developmental Disabilities.* Eastman, QC, Canada: Diverse City Press.

Janz, Tom, and Mooney, Greg. (1991). *Behavior Description Interviewing: Trainer's Package.* Frenchs Forest, NSW, Australia: Pearson Education Australia.

Jinkins, Michael, and Jinkins, Deborah Bradshaw. (1998). *The Character of Leadership: Political Realism and Public Virtue in Nonprofit Organizations.* San Francisco: Jossey-Bass.

Kraft, Alisa Hauser. (2002). *Feel Our Freedom: Communities and Connections for People with Developmental Disabilities.* Homewood, IL: High Tide Press.

Kunc, Norman, and Van der Klift, Emma. (1996). *A Credo for Support* [Video-tape]. Nanaimo, BC, Canada: Axis Consultation & Training.

Lovett, Herbert. (1996). *Learning to Listen: Positive Approaches and People with Difficult Behavior.* Baltimore: Paul H. Brookes.

Luiselli, James K., and Cameron, Michael J. (1998). *Antecedent Control: Innovative Approaches to Behavioral Support.* Baltimore: Paul H. Brookes.

McCartney, John R., and Campbell, Vincent A. (1988). Confirmed Abuse Cases in Public Residential Facilities for Persons with Mental Retardation: A Multi-State Study. *Mental Retardation* 36 (6), 465-473.

McNamara, Roger. *Not Knowingly Do Harm* [On-line]. No longer available: www.freedomfromabuse.org.

Mercer, Mary. (2003). *Person-Centered Planning: Helping People with Disabilities Achieve Personal Outcomes.* Homewood, IL: High Tide Press.

Money Smart–An Adult Education Program. Washington, DC: Federal Deposit Insurance Corporation.

Murray, Les. (1992). "Dog Fox Field" from *Dog Fox Field: Poems.* New York: Farrar Straus & Giroux.

Mount, B., and Zwernik, K. (1988). *It's Never Too Early, It's Never Too Late: A Booklet about Personal Futures Planning.* St. Paul, MN: Metropolitan Council.

Nelson, Bob, and Blanchard, Kenneth. (1994). *1001 Ways to Reward Employees.* New York: Workman.

Crisis Prevention Institute. (2004). *Instructor Manual for the Nonviolent Crisis Intervention[R] Training Program.* Brookfield, WI: Author.

North Dakota Center for Persons with Disabilities. (2003). *Guidebook for QMRPs.* Minot, ND: Author.

Pomeranz, Tom. (2001). *The Principles and Practices of Universal Enhancement. Vol. 1: It Matters How We Say It.* Homewood, IL: High Tide Press.

Pryor, Karen. (1999). *Don't Shoot the Dog: The New Art of Teaching and Training.* New York: Bantam.

Ray, Nancy K. (2000). *Abuse and Neglect Prevention in Community Homes*. Presentation at Illinois American Association on Mental Retardation Conference, Collinsville, IL.

Reid, Dennis H., Parsons, Marsha B., and Green, Carolyn W. (1989). *Staff Management in Human Services: Behavioral Research and Applications*. Springfield, IL: Charles E. Thomas.

Research and Training Center on Community Living, (2004). *Direct Support: A Realistic Job Preview* [Video]. (Available at Research Training Center of Community Living, University of Minnesota, Minneapolis, MN).

Reynolds, Leigh Ann. (2001). *People with Mental Retardation and Sexual Abuse. The ARC's Q & A on People with Mental Retardation*. [On-line]. Available: from www.thearc.org/faqs/Sexabuse.html (accessed July 7, 2005).

Rivera, Geraldo. (Producer and director). (1972). *Unforgotten: 25 Years after Willowbrook* [Video]. (Available at Program Development Associates, P. O. Box 2038, Syracuse, NY 13220-2038).

Self Advocates Becoming Empowered (SABE), http://www.sabe.org.

Shephard, John. (2001). *The Suzie Brown Intervention Maze*. Homewood, IL: High Tide Press.

Sobsey, Dick. (1994). *Violence and Abuse in the Lives of People with Disabilities: The End of Silent Acceptance?* Baltimore: Paul H. Brookes.

Spector, Paul E. (1997). *Job Satisfaction: Application, Assessment, Causes and Consequences*. Thousand Oaks, CA: Sage.

Suess, George. (2000). *Shift Happens: Making the Shift to Proactive Behavior Management*. Walton, NY: Delaware County Arc.

Townsley, Ruth, et al. (1996). *Getting Involved in Choosing Staff: A Resource Pack for Supporters, Trainers, and Staff Working with People Who Have Developmental Disabilities.* Bristol, England: Policy Press.

Tyler, Carl. (1999). *Medical Issues for Adults with Mental Retardation/Developmental Disabilities.* Homewood, IL: High Tide Press.

Walker-Hirsch, Leslie, and Champagne, Marklyn P. (1993). *Circles I: Intimacy & Relationships.* Santa Barbara, CA: James Stanfield.

Weick, Carl, and Sutcliffe, Kathleen M. (2001). *Managing the Unexpected.* San Francisco: Jossey-Bass.

Wiseman, Frederick. (1967). *Titticut Follies* [Video]. (Available from Zipporah Films, Inc., 1 Richdale Avenue, Unit 4, Cambridge, MA 02140).

Appendices

Appendix A: Operational Definitions for People Supported Worksheet

Appendix B: Operational Definitions for Paid Staff Worksheet

Appendix C: People Supported Data Sheet

Appendix D: Paid Staff Data Sheet

Appendix E: Recording Data Quick Reference Guide

Appendix A - Page 1
Operational Definitions for People Supported Worksheet

Key Indicator		Operational Definitions	Data Sources
P-1	History of Abuse/Neglect/Exploitation		
P-2	Reputation		
P-3	Involved Medical Care		
P-4	Involved Personal Care		
P-5	Behavioral Issues		

Appendix A - Page 2
Operational Definitions for People Supported Worksheet

Key Indicator		Operational Definitions	Data Sources
P-6	Fiscal vulnerability		
P-7	Empowerment		
P-8	Down Time		
P-9	Satisfaction		
P-10	Individual Service Plan		

Appendix B - Page 1
Operational Definitions for Paid Staff Worksheet

Key Indicator		Operational Definitions	Data Sources
S-1	Vulnerability		
S-2	Integrity		
S-3	Isolation		
S-4	Competence		
S-5	Confidence		

Appendix B - Page 2
Operational Definitions for Paid Staff Worksheet

Key Indicator		Operational Definitions	Data Sources
S-6	Voice/Language		
S-7	Overtime		
S-8	Job Satisfaction		
S-9	Supervisor Relationship		
S-10	Employee Feedback		

Appendix C: People Supported Data Sheet

Date: _____   Reviewer: _____   Location: _____

Person Supported	P-1	P-2	P-3	P-4	P-5	P-6	P-7	P-8	P-9	P-10	Total
Total											
%											

Appendix D: Paid Staff Data Sheet

Date: _____   Reviewer: _____   Location: _____

Paid Staff	S-1	S-2	S-3	S-4	S-5	S-6	S-7	S-8	S-9	S-10	Total
Total											
%											

Appendix E
Data Recording Quick Reference Guide

Issue		Operational Definitions	Data Sources
People Supported Domain Issues			
P1	History of Abuse & Neglect		
P2	Reputation		
P3	Involved Medical Care		
P4	Involved Personal Care		
P5	Behavioral Issues/Plans		
P6	Fiscal Vulnerability		
P7	Individual Empowerment		
P8	Down Time		
P9	Satisfaction		
P10	Individual Service Plan		
Paid Staff Domain Issues			
S1	Vulnerability		
S2	Integrity		
S3	Isolation		
S4	Competence		
S5	Confidence		
S6	Voice/Language		
S7	Overtime		
S8	Job Satisfaction		
S9	Supervisor Relationship		
S10	Employee Feedback		

About the Authors

Steve Baker accidentally fell into working for service provider agencies while looking for a part-time job in college. Since then, he has managed nearly every aspect of service organizations for people with intellectual disabilities. Currently, he works as a program director at Trinity Services, Inc. in Joliet, IL. He is also the Executive Director of The Midewin Institute, a partnership dedicated to the prevention of abuse and neglect of adults with mental disabilities.

Mr. Baker holds a master's degree in psychology from the University of Nevada-Reno. He can be reached via e-mail at sbaker@trinity-services.org.

Amy Tabor began her career working in a group home for individuals with autism and has since held a variety of roles within human service agencies. Now, as the President of Organizational Dimensions, Ms. Tabor leads the consulting firm in developing resources for nonprofits. The firm specializes in staff training, quality enhancement and organizational improvement. Ms. Tabor holds undergraduate and graduate degrees in sociology and regularly presents at conferences across the nation. Ms. Tabor resides with her husband, Jim, and their three children in Fairhope, AL. She can be reached via e-mail at aetabor@bellsouth.net or OrganizDim@aol.com.

Mr. Baker and Ms. Tabor have collaborated on a number of projects, including the monograph *Human Rights Committees: Keeping Organizations on Course* (High Tide Press, 1999). Now in its third edition, the book has also been translated into Japanese and Chinese. Readers are invited to contact the authors with questions and comments.